A HEALTHY MINDSET:
TRACKER & ACTIVITY WORKBOOK FOR KIDS

SAVOR EDUCATION

NUTRITION BY DESIGN

WWW.SAVOREDUCATION.COM

A HEALTHY MINDSET:
TRACKER & ACTIVITY WORKBOOK FOR KIDS

Four Week Super Health Challenge

What is MyPlate?

MyPlate is the communication tool the U.S. government uses to share the Dietary Guidelines for Americans with the general public. The Dietary Guidelines for Americans provide advice on what to eat and drink to meet nutrient needs, promote health and prevent disease. This workbook and tracker are designed in accordance with the 2020-2025 Dietary Guidelines and provide a customizable framework for healthy eating and activity choices.

Week 1

Review the five food groups and consider the importance of having a variety of foods from all five food groups. Consider why each food group is uniquely important.

Complete the following:

All About Healthy Me
Week 1 Road to Health Goals
Super Health Tracker

Week 2

Complete the following:

Match the Food to the Food Group
Coloring My Plate
Week 2 - Road to Health Goals
Super Health Tracker

Week 3

Complete the following:

My Body Needs Table
What Counts Worksheet
Week 3 - Road to Health Goals
Super Health Tracker

Week 4

Complete the following:

Connections - Food and Body
Food and Nutrients
Essential Nutrients Word Search
Week 4 - Road to Health Goals
Super Health Tracker
Super Health Challenge Certificate of Completion

Fruit Group

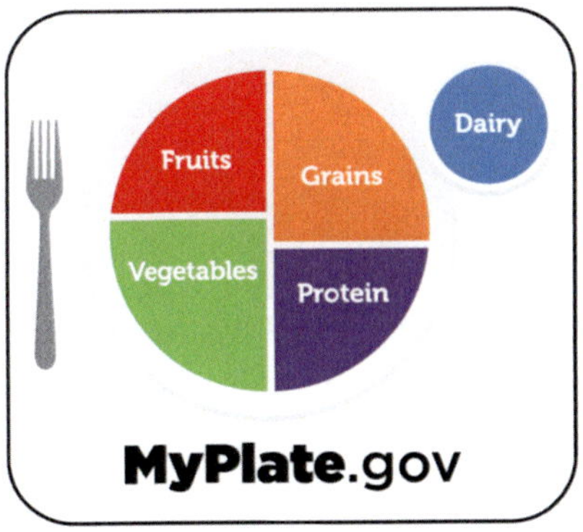

The fruit group includes fresh, frozen, canned and dried fruits. Fruits can be eaten whole, sliced, puréed or consumed as 100% fruit juices. Fruits are naturally high in fiber, potassium, folate and vitamin C.

Focus On Fruits

These essential nutrients benefit your body:

Fiber: benefits our bodies in many ways. Fiber-containing foods, like fruits, help your body feel full and benefit our gut microbiome by fueling the healthy bacteria in our bodies! Fiber also reduces the risk of heart disease by lowering cholesterol levels in our blood keeping vessels free of clots.

Potassium: regulates the fluid inside and outside of our cells ensuring the normal functioning of all the cells in our bodies. It helps regulate our heartbeat and is vital for creating proteins and using carbohydrates for fuel.

Folate: is important in red blood cell formation as well as healthy cell growth and function. This nutrient is crucial during early pregnancy to reduce the risk of birth defects.

Vitamin C: supports healing cuts and wounds, grows, and repairs body tissues, and maintains healthy teeth and gums.

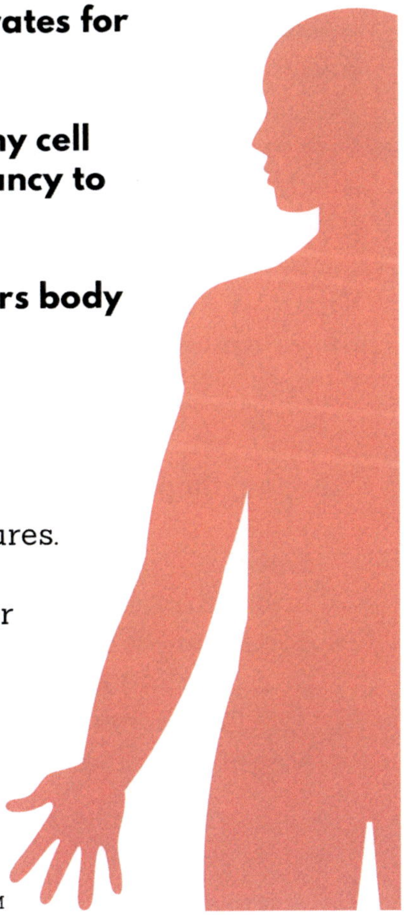

Tips for choosing foods from the fruit group:

- Choose a variety of fruit in a rainbow of colors, flavors, and textures.
- Choose canned fruit packed in water or 100% juice.
- Juice should be 100% fruit juice for lower added sugar and higher nutrient content.
- Fruits are great for breakfast, lunch, dinner and dessert.
- Ripe fruit can be frozen and added to smoothies.
- Keep fruit handy for an on-the-go snack.

Vegetable Group

The vegetable group includes fresh, frozen, and canned veggies. Vegetables are naturally high in Fiber, Potassium, Vitamin E and Vitamin A.

Vary Your Veggies

These essential nutrients benefit your body:

Fiber: benefits our bodies in many ways. Fiber-containing foods, like vegetables, help your body feel full and benefit our gut microbiome by fueling the healthy bacteria in our bodies! Fiber also reduces the risk of heart disease by lowering cholesterol levels in our blood keeping vessels free of clots.

Potassium: regulates the fluid inside and outside of our cells ensuring the normal functioning of all the cells in our bodies. It helps regulate our heartbeat, is vital for creating proteins, and using carbohydrates for fuel.

Vitamin E: role in the body is to act as an antioxidant, scavenging loose electrons or "free radicals" that can damage cells. It also enhances immune function and prevents clots from forming in arteries.

Vitamin A: supports normal cell growth, immune function, and vision. It plays an important role in healthy fetal development.

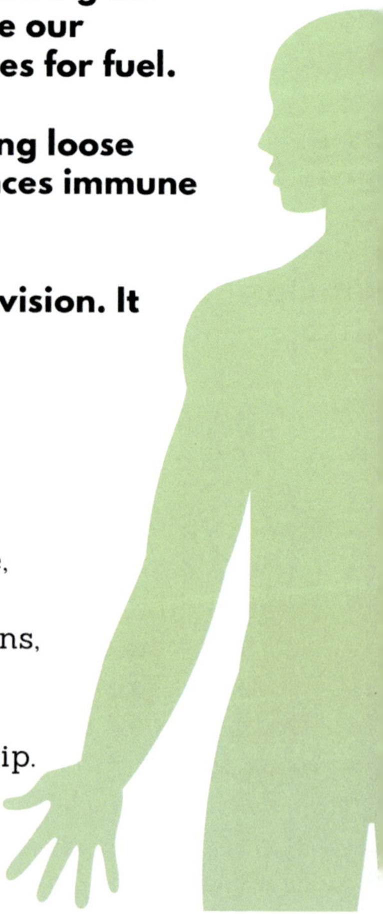

Tips for choosing foods from the vegetable group:

- Choose a variety of vegetables including dark green, red, orange, and starchy.
- Fresh and frozen veggies are an excellent source of fiber, vitamins, and nutrients.
- Try beans, peas or lentils for a boost of vegetable protein.
- Vegetables make a perfect snack. Try them with your favorite dip.

Grains Group

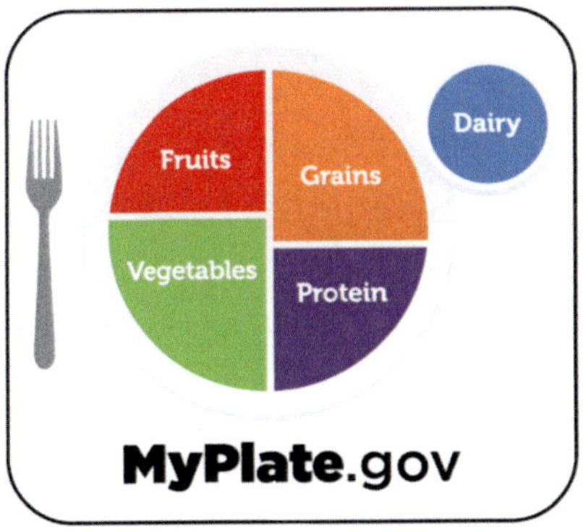

Grain group foods include any product made from wheat, oats, cornmeal, barley, or another cereal grain. Grains are an important source of fiber and several B vitamins (thiamin, riboflavin and niacin)

Make Half Your Grains Whole Grains

These essential nutrients benefit your body:

Fiber: benefits our bodies in many ways. Fiber-containing foods, like vegetables, help your body feel full and benefit our gut microbiome by fueling the healthy bacteria in our bodies! Fiber also reduces the risk of heart disease by lowering cholesterol levels in our blood keeping vessels free of clots.

Thiamin: helps our bodies convert nutrients, like carbohydrates, into energy. This energy metabolism makes growth, development, and cell function possible while keeping your nervous system healthy.

Riboflavin: is essential for many body processes. The development of skin and the lining of your digestive tract is one of those processes. It is also necessary for the function of your brain and blood cells.

Niacin: plays an important role in lowering cholesterol in your blood and assists in converting food and nutrients into energy.

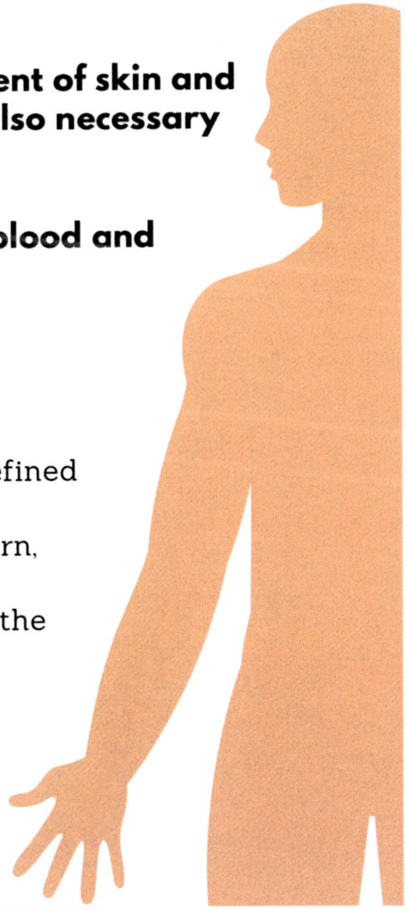

Tips for choosing foods from the grains group:

- A whole grain, in general, contains more fiber and nutrients than refined grain.
- Try new whole-grain foods like brown rice, oats, corn, barley, popcorn, farro, and quinoa.
- Did you know? All whole grain is made up of three parts: the bran, the germ and the endosperm.
- The term "whole-grain" is used on packaging and means that the product contains all three portions of the kernel (bran, germ and endosperm.)

Dairy Group

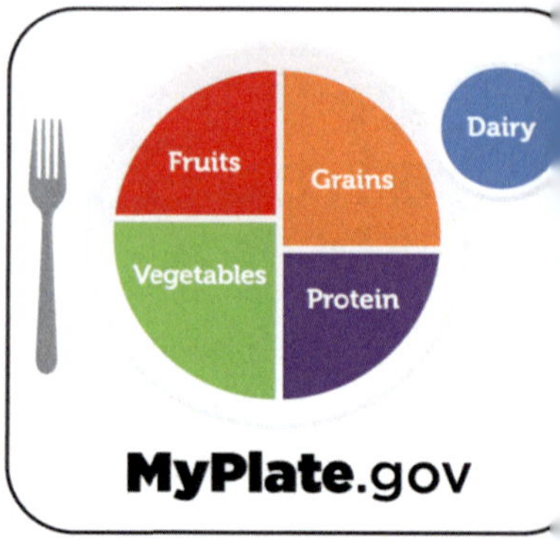

Dairy foods include milk, yogurt, cheese, lactose-free milk and fortified soy milk and yogurt. It does not include foods made from milk that have little calcium and high-fat content like cream cheese, sour cream, cream and butter.

Move to Low-fat or Fat-free Dairy Milk or Yogurt

These essential nutrients benefit your body:

Calcium: is needed for building and maintaining strong bones and teeth at all ages. Calcium also plays a role in regulating normal heart rhythms and nerve function.

Vitamin D: has many functions in the body but plays an important role in the body's ability to absorb and retain calcium and phosphorus needed for bones, growth and the repair of tissues.

Phosphorus: in addition to maintaining strong bones and teeth, phosphorus is needed for the production of your genetic building blocks, DNA and RNA.

Potassium: regulates the fluid inside and outside of our cells ensuring the normal functioning of all the cells in our bodies. It helps regulate our heartbeat, is vital for creating proteins, and using carbohydrates for fuel.

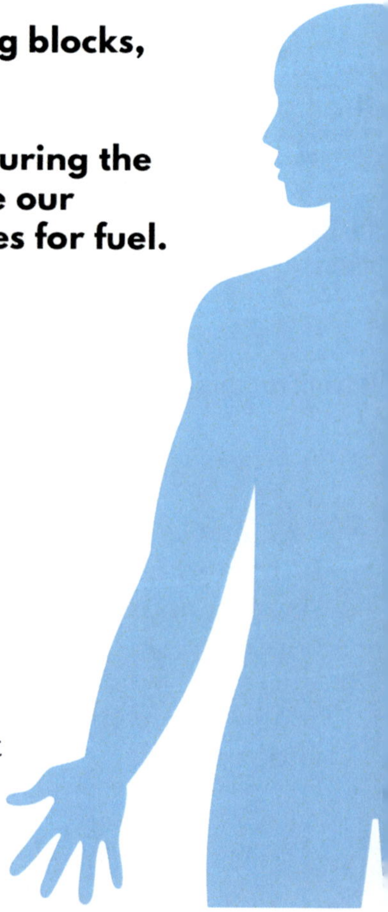

Tips for choosing foods from the dairy group:

- Choose low-fat or skim milk. Low-fat contains less than 1% milk fat. Skim milk, is less than .5% milk fat.
- Try fermented dairy products like yogurt and kefir to boost digestive health.
- Dairy alternatives, fortified soy milk and yogurt have calcium, vitamin A and vitamin D added. This is why these products are included in the dairy group because their nutrient content is comparable to dairy milk and yogurt.
- Other products served as "milk" may contain calcium, but are not part of the dairy group because their content is not comparable to dairy milk or yogurt.

Protein Foods Group

All foods made from seafood, meat, poultry, eggs, nuts, seeds and soy products are part of the protein foods group. Beans, peas and lentils are part of both the protein foods group and the vegetable food group.

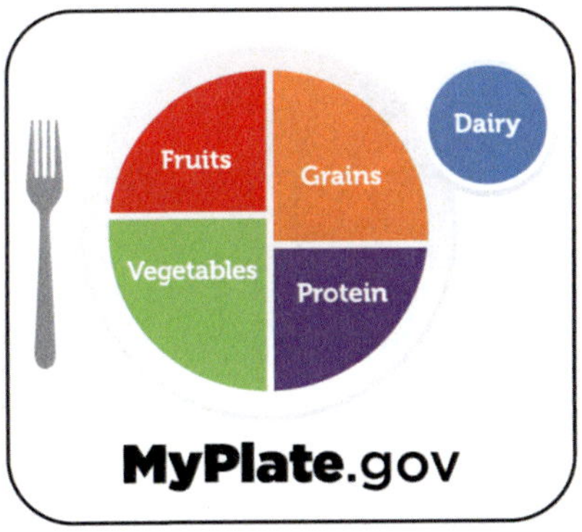

Vary Your Protein Routine

These essential nutrients benefit your body:

Proteins: are essential building blocks for the structure, function and regulation of your body systems. Your blood, bones, muscle, cartilage and skin are all built from proteins. Protein is also one of three nutrients that provide calories or energy (the others are fat and carbohydrates.)

Iron: is important because it allows your blood to transport oxygen from your lungs to your body tissues.

Zinc: supports a healthy immune system by fighting off invading viruses and bacteria. It also helps nerves carry messages between the brain and the body.

Magnesium: is needed for more than 300 biochemical enzyme reactions in the body. It is needed to support muscle and nerve function.

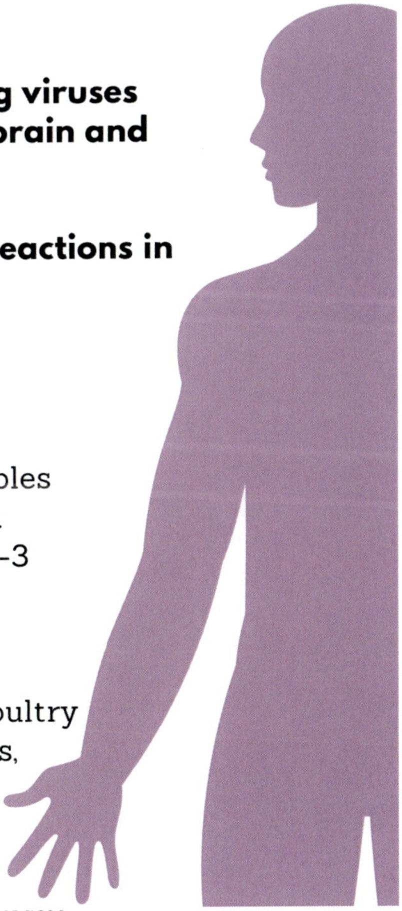

Tips for choosing foods from the protein food group:

- Choose meat and poultry choices that are lean or low-fat. Examples include lean ground beef, pork loin, and skinless chicken breasts.
- Try to have seafood like salmon or trout once a week for omega-3 fatty acids that support heart health.
- Plant-forward meals can still contain complete proteins like the combination of beans and rice.
- Most Americans meet the protein recommendations for meat, poultry and eggs but do not meet the recommendations for seafood, nuts, seeds and soy products.

All About Healthy Me

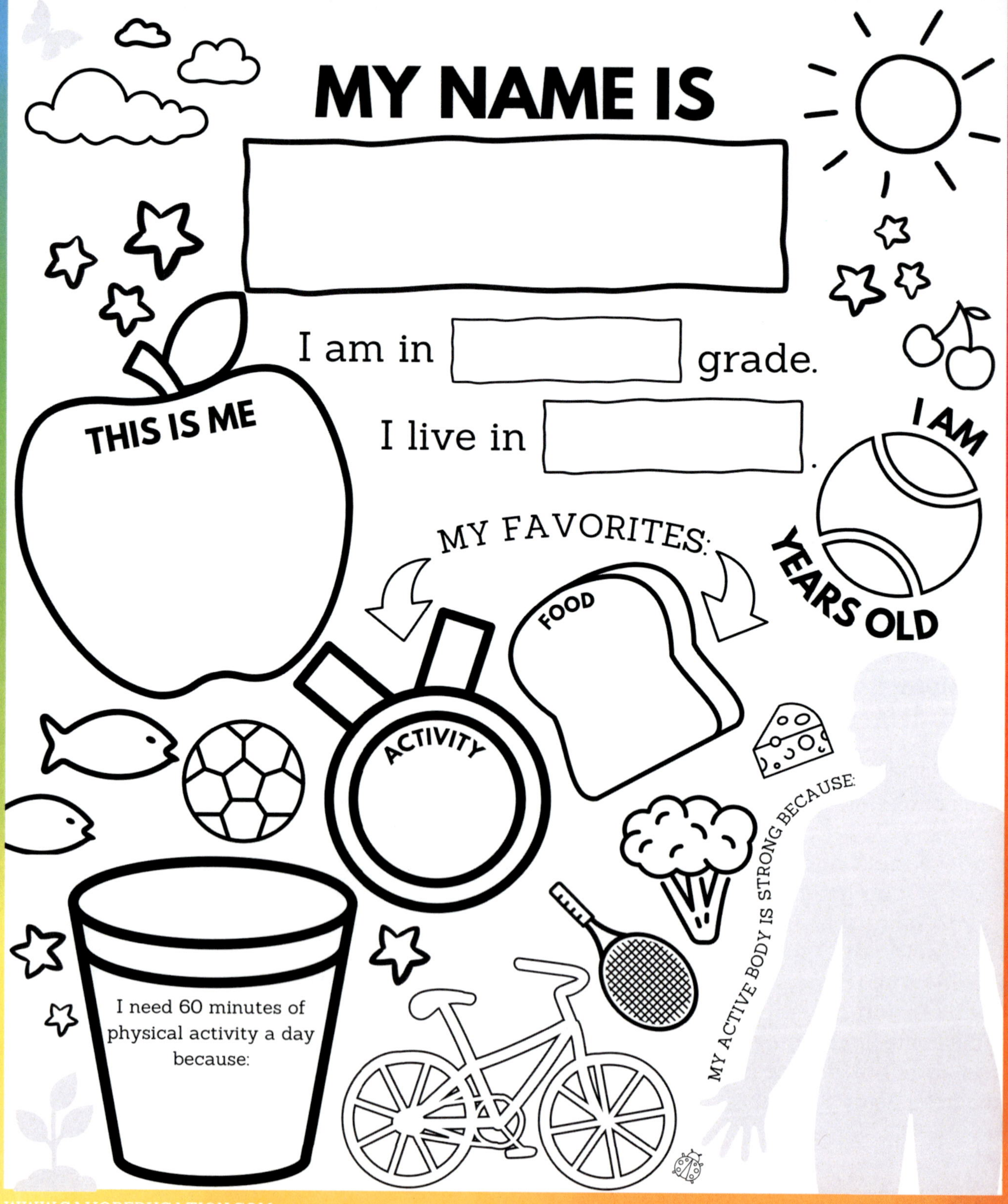

Match the Foods to the Food Group

NAME:

DRAW A LINE FROM THE FOOD TO THE MYPLATE FOOD GROUP YOU THINK IT BELONGS.

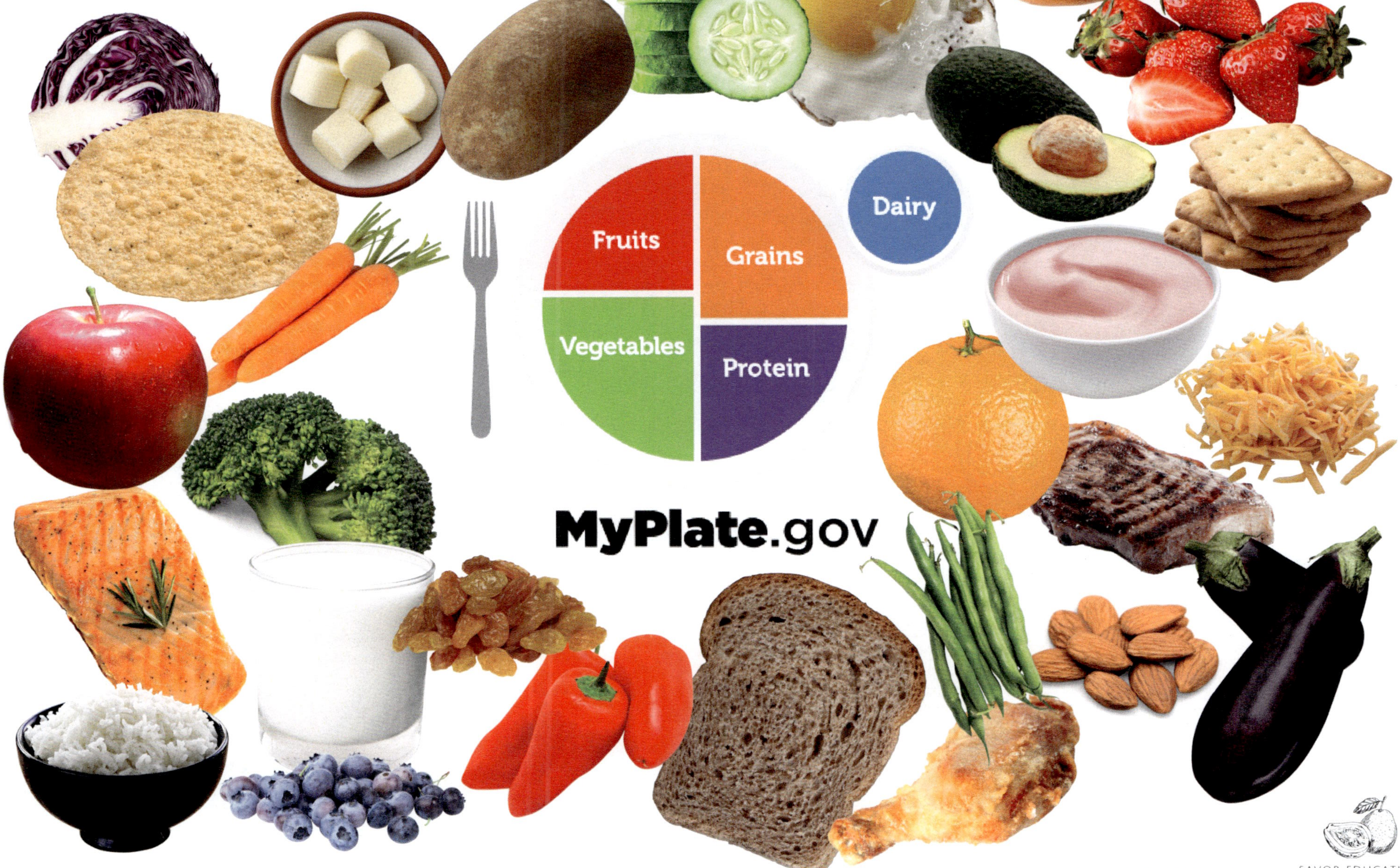

WWW.SAVOREDUCATION.COM

SAVOR EDUCATION
NUTRITION BY DESIGN

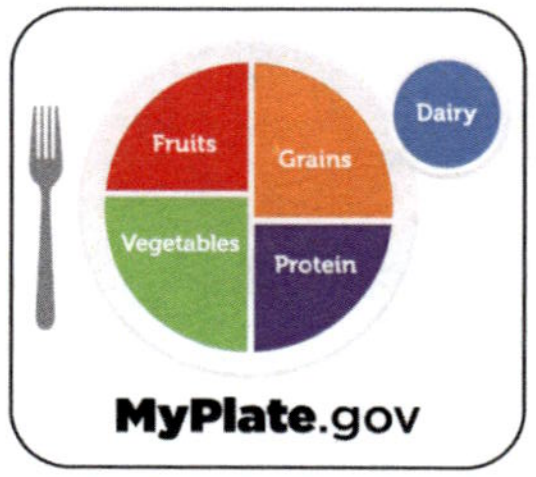

Coloring My Plate

DRAW THE FOODS YOU ENJOY IN EACH FOOD GROUP.

NAME:

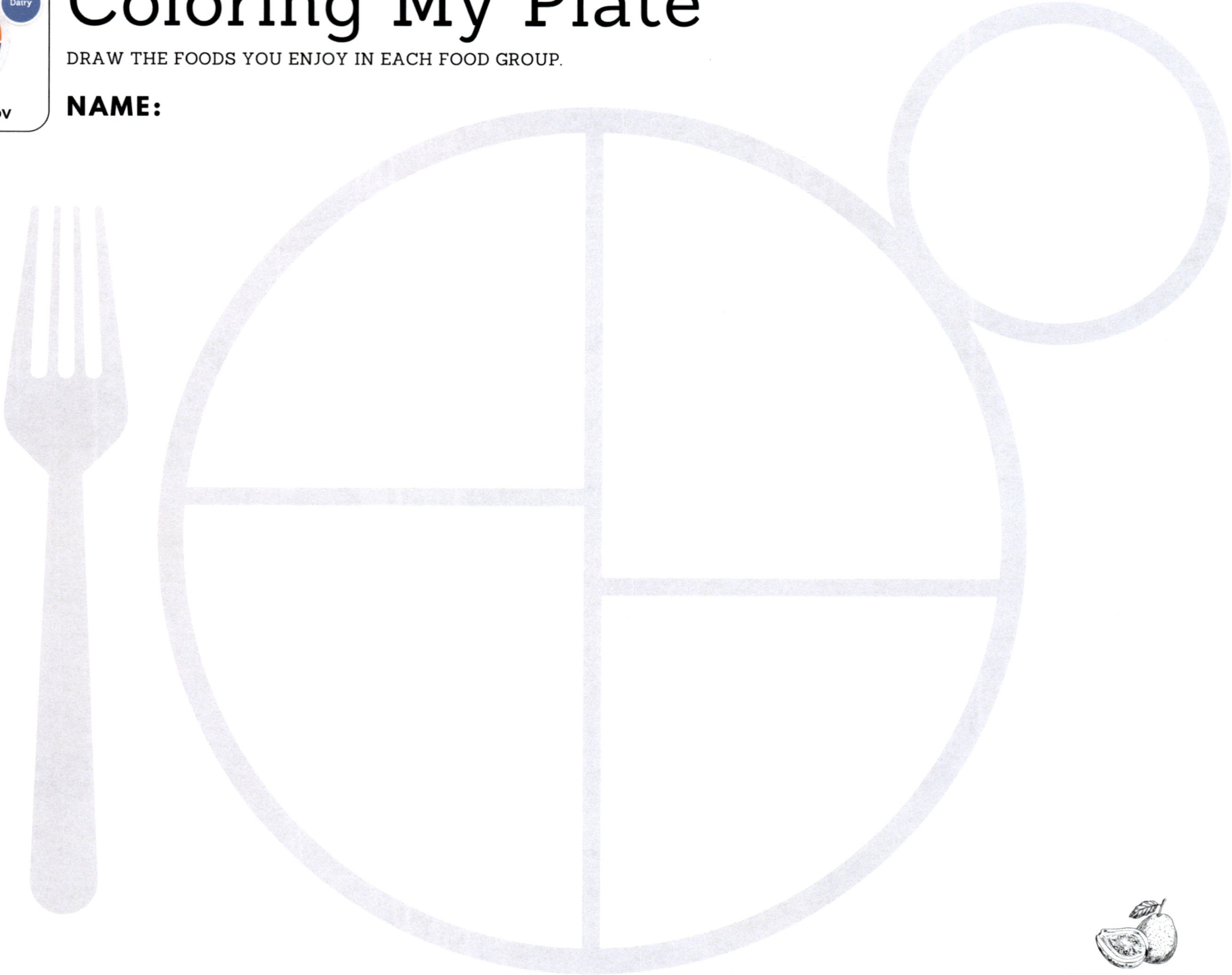

WWW.SAVOREDUCATION.COM

SAVOR EDUCATION
NUTRITION BY DESIGN

My Body Needs Table

DAILY RECOMMENDATIONS*

CIRCLE YOUR AGE GROUP BELOW. NEXT, CIRCLE THE COLUMN BELOW YOUR AGE GROUP. THIS IS THE AMOUNT YOUR BODY NEEDS FROM EACH FOOD GROUP.

HOW MUCH EQUALS A CUP OR AN OUNCE?

Food Group	Children 5- 8	Girls 9-13	Boys 9-13	Cup and Ounce Equivalents
Fruits FOCUS ON WHOLE FRUITS	1 to 2 cups	1 1/2 to 2 cups	1 1/2 to 2 cups	1 cup fresh or frozen 1/2 cup dried 1 cup 100% fruit juice (6 oz per day for kids 6 years and younger)
Vegetables VARY YOUR VEGGIES	1 1/2 to 2 1/2 cups	1 1/2 to 3 cups	2 to 3 1/2 cups	1 cup raw or cooked 2 cups raw leafy greens
Grains MAKE HALF YOUR GRAINS WHOLE	4 to 6 oz equiv	5 to 7 oz equiv	5 to 9 oz equiv	One slice of bread 1/2 cup cooked pasta, rice or grain 1 cup dry cold cereal
Protein Foods VARY YOUR PROTEIN ROUTINE	3 to 5 1/2 oz equiv	4 to 6 oz equiv	5 to 6 1/2 oz equiv	1 oz cooked lean meat 1 egg 1/4 cup cooked beans or lentils 1 Tbsp nut butter and 1/2 oz nuts
Dairy MOVE TO LOW-FAT OR FAT-FREE MILK OR YOGURT	2 1/2 cups	3 cups	3 cups	1 cup milk or yogurt 1 1/2 ounces hard cheese 1/3 cup shredded cheese

• THESE ARE GENERAL RECOMMENDATIONS

What Counts?

1. USING THE COLUMN YOU CIRCLED ON THE "MY BODY NEEDS TABLE," FILL IN THE BLANK FOR THE AMOUNTS YOU NEED FROM EACH FOOD GROUP BELOW.
2. CIRCLE THE FOODS THAT EQUAL THE NUMBER OF DAILY CUP OR OUNCE EQUIVALENTS YOUR BODY NEEDS.

Fruit

- 8 STRAWBERRIES = 1 CUP
- 1 CUP BLUEBERRIES = 1 CUP
- 1 CUP 100% JUICE = 1 CUP
- 1 LARGE APPLE = 1 CUP
- 1/2 CUP DRIED FRUIT = 1 CUP
- 1 LARGE BANANA = 1 CUP
- 1 LARGE ORANGE = 1 CUP

Daily Cups of Fruit I Need ____

Vegetable

- 6 BABY CARROTS = 1 CUP
- 1 CUP COOKED = 1 CUP
- 1 MEDIUM POTATO = 1 CUP
- 2 CUPS LETTUCE = 1 CUP
- 3 SMALL PEPPERS = 1 CUP
- 8 CUCUMBER SLICES = 1 CUP
- 1 CUP BROCCOLI = 1 CUP

Daily Cups of Vegetables I Need ____

Grain

- 1/2 CUP COOKED RICE = 1 OUNCE
- 7 CRACKERS = 1 OUNCE
- 1 - 6 INCH TORTILLA = 1 OUNCE
- 1 CUP COOKED CEREAL = 1 OUNCE
- 1 SLICE OF BREAD = 1 OUNCE
- 1 CUP READY - TO-EAT CEREAL = 1 OUNCE

Daily Ounces of Grains I Need ____

Protein Foods

- 1 OUNCE CHICKEN = 1 OUNCE
- 1 EGG = 1 OUNCE
- 12 ALMONDS = 1 OUNCE
- 1 OUNCE SALMON = 1 OUNCE
- 1/4 CUP COOKED BEANS = 1 OUNCE
- 1 OUNCE HAMBURGER = 1 OUNCE

Daily Ounces of Protein Foods I Need ____

Dairy

- 1 1/2 OUNCES HARD CHEESE = 1 CUP
- 1 CUP MILK = 1 CUP
- 1 SCHOOL MILK = 1 CUP
- 1 CUP YOGURT = 1 CUP
- 1/3 CUP SHREDDED CHEESE = 1 CUP
- 2 CUPS COTTAGE CHEESE = 1 CUP

Daily Cups of Dairy I Need

Connections Food & Body

MAKE THE CONNECTION BETWEEN THE FOODS AND THE NUTRIENTS THEY CONTAIN. EACH FOOD CONTAINS NUTRIENTS THAT PLAY A ROLE IN KEEPING YOUR BODY HEALTHY.
DRAW THE BODY PART ON THE BODY BELOW AND A LINE TO THE NUTRIENT AND FOODS THAT KEEP IT HEALTHY.

NAME:

Potassium

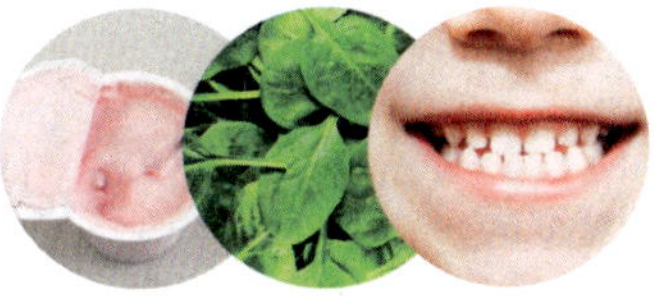

Protein

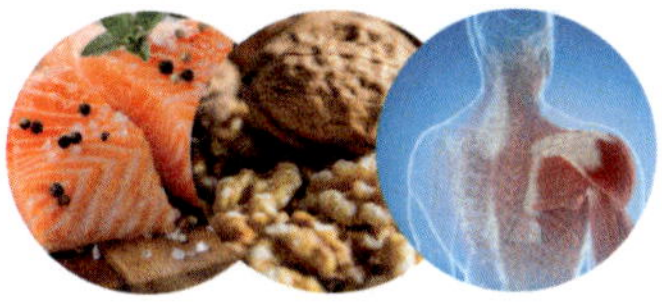

Vitamin E

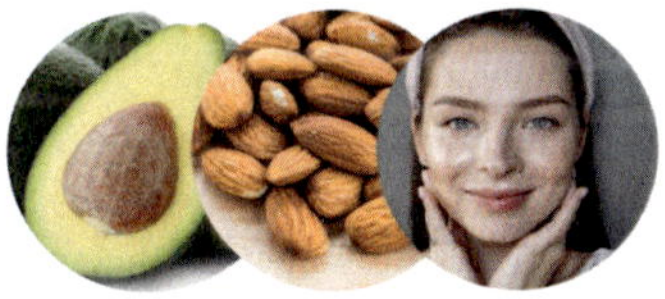

Iron

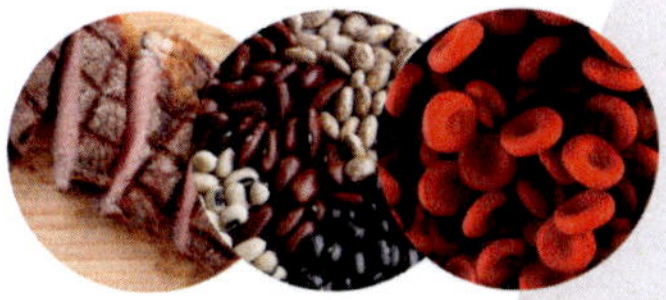

Vitamin D

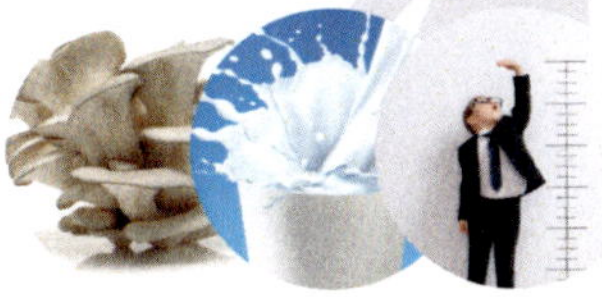

Vitamin A

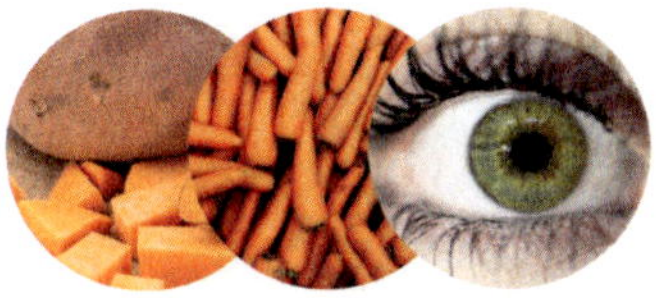

Calcium

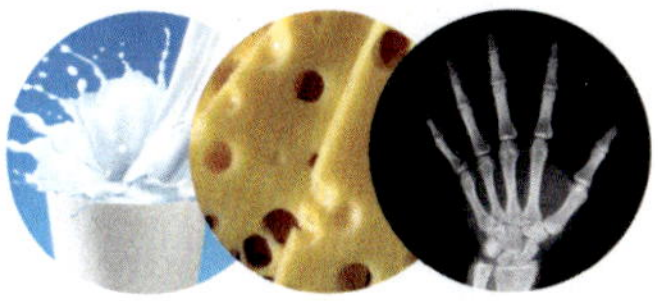

Thiamin

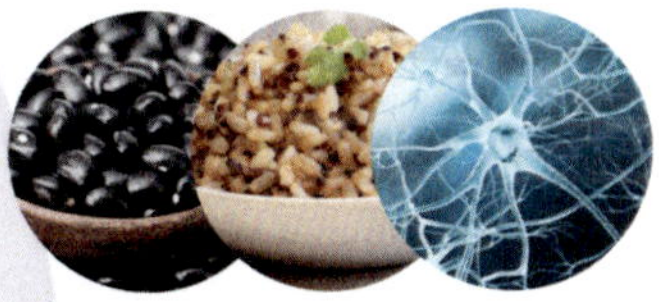

Vitamin C

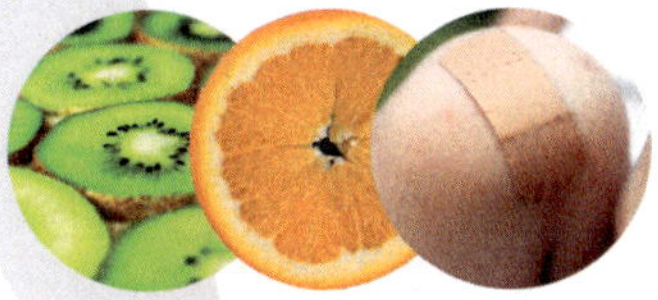

Fiber

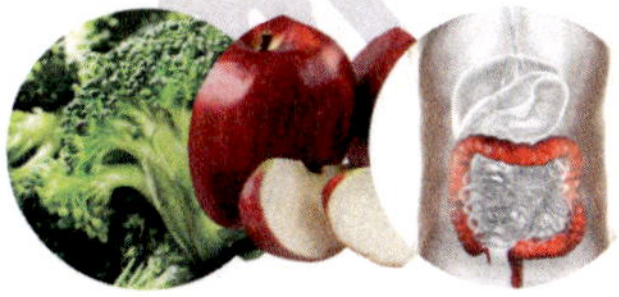

Foods and Nutrients

NAME:

1. ALL THE FOODS BELOW ARE GOOD SOURCES OF AT LEAST ONE ESSENTIAL NUTRIENT. DRAW A LINE FROM THE FOOD TO THE NUTRIENTS YOU THINK THAT FOOD MAY CONTAIN. DIFFERENT FOOD GROUPS CONTAIN DIFFERENT NUTRIENTS. USE THE COLOR OF THE BOX AROUND THE NUTRIENT AS A CLUE.
2. WRITE WHY YOU THINK IT IS IMPORTANT TO CHOOSE FOODS FROM ALL FIVE FOOD GROUPS AT THE BOTTOM OF THE PAGE.

FIBER | VITAMIN C | CALCIUM | IRON | POTASSIUM | PROTEIN | VITAMIN A | THIAMIN

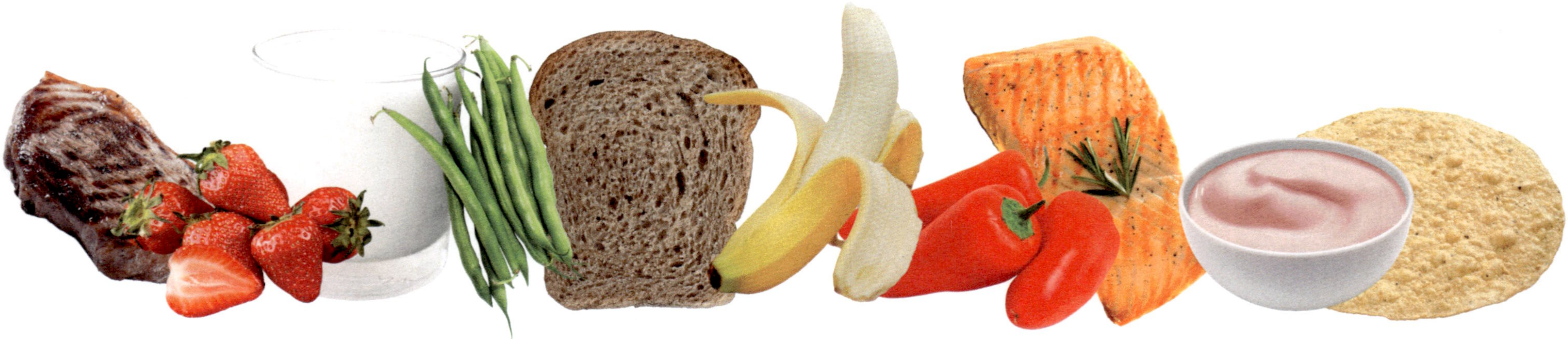

Essential Nutrients Word Search

NAME:

CIRCLE AS MANY NUTRIENTS AS YOU CAN FIND.

FIND THE FOLLOWING WORDS IN THE PUZZLE. WORDS ARE HIDDEN ⇨ ⇩ AND ⇘

P	C	N	G	J	H	P	R	E	V	I	T	A	M	I	N	A	M
M	A	A	X	H	T	H	R	I	P	I	X	C	J	D	X	R	A
Y	L	V	R	X	Q	O	Y	P	B	O	T	Q	Z	R	N	Q	G
F	C	I	L	B	A	S	U	G	R	O	T	A	P	I	E	G	N
I	I	T	I	Q	O	P	T	J	N	O	F	A	M	C	N	B	E
B	U	A	R	G	S	H	F	H	P	M	T	L	S	I	M	C	S
E	M	M	O	T	X	O	Y	U	I	W	O	E	A	S	N	R	I
R	B	I	N	V	H	R	Z	D	Y	A	G	H	I	V	I	D	U
L	Q	N	D	O	O	U	L	J	R	Q	M	F	B	N	I	U	M
X	K	B	L	N	E	S	V	I	T	A	M	I	N	E	Q	N	M
M	R	L	F	O	L	A	T	E	Q	D	T	D	N	G	P	U	Y
N	I	A	C	I	N	D	L	Y	I	O	R	E	H	F	P	S	S

FIBER
IRON
POTASSIUM
FOLATE
THIAMIN
RIBOFLAVIN
NIACIN
VITAMIN A
VITAMIN B
CALCIUM
VITAMIN D
VITAMIN E
ZINC
MAGNESIUM
PHOSPHORUS
CARBOHYDRATE
PROTEIN

Road to Health Goals:

NAME:

WEEK 1

Be active!
I intend to:

Choose
nutrient-rich foods!
I intend to:

Challenges
I might face:

Super Health Tracker

NAME:

TRACK THE DAILY SERVINGS YOU EAT FROM EACH FOOD GROUP AND LOG YOUR ACTIVITY. FINDING ACTIVITIES YOU ENJOY AND CHOOSING A VARIETY OF FOODS FROM ALL FIVE FOOD GROUPS HELPS YOU GROW HEALTHY AND STRONG! DRAW OR WRITE YOUR FAVORITE FOOD YOU CHOSE FROM THAT FOOD GROUP WHERE INDICATED BELOW.

MyPlate.gov

	FRUIT GROUP FOODS I ATE:	VEGETABLE GROUP FOODS I ATE:	GRAIN GROUP FOODS I ATE:	PROTEIN GROUP FOODS I ATE:	DAIRY GROUP FOODS I ATE:
MONDAY DO YOUR ACTIVITES = 60 MINUTES? ☐ YES	☐☐☐☐☐ MY FAVORITE FRUIT:	☐☐☐☐☐ MY FAVORITE VEGGIE:	☐☐☐☐☐ MY FAVORITE GRAIN:	☐☐☐☐☐ MY FAVORITE PROTEIN:	☐☐☐☐☐ MY FAVORITE DAIRY:
TUESDAY DO YOUR ACTIVITES = 60 MINUTES? ☐ YES	☐☐☐☐☐ MY FAVORITE FRUIT:	☐☐☐☐☐ MY FAVORITE VEGGIE:	☐☐☐☐☐ MY FAVORITE GRAIN:	☐☐☐☐☐ MY FAVORITE PROTEIN:	☐☐☐☐☐ MY FAVORITE DAIRY:
WEDNESDAY DO YOUR ACTIVITES = 60 MINUTES? ☐ YES	☐☐☐☐☐ MY FAVORITE FRUIT:	☐☐☐☐☐ MY FAVORITE VEGGIE:	☐☐☐☐☐ MY FAVORITE GRAIN:	☐☐☐☐☐ MY FAVORITE PROTEIN:	☐☐☐☐☐ MY FAVORITE DAIRY:
THURSDAY DO YOUR ACTIVITES = 60 MINUTES? ☐ YES	☐☐☐☐☐ MY FAVORITE FRUIT:	☐☐☐☐☐ MY FAVORITE VEGGIE:	☐☐☐☐☐ MY FAVORITE GRAIN:	☐☐☐☐☐ MY FAVORITE PROTEIN:	☐☐☐☐☐ MY FAVORITE DAIRY:
FRIDAY DO YOUR ACTIVITES = 60 MINUTES? ☐ YES	☐☐☐☐☐ MY FAVORITE FRUIT:	☐☐☐☐☐ MY FAVORITE VEGGIE:	☐☐☐☐☐ MY FAVORITE GRAIN:	☐☐☐☐☐ MY FAVORITE PROTEIN:	☐☐☐☐☐ MY FAVORITE DAIRY:

SAVOR EDUCATION
NUTRITION BY DESIGN

Road to Health Goals:

NAME:

WEEK 2

Be active!
I intend to:

____
____
____
____
____
____

Choose
nutrient-rich foods!
I intend to:

____
____
____
____
____
____

Challenges
I might face:

____
____
____
____
____
____

Super Health Tracker

NAME:

TRACK THE DAILY SERVINGS YOU EAT FROM EACH FOOD GROUP AND LOG YOUR ACTIVITY. FINDING ACTIVITIES YOU ENJOY AND CHOOSING A VARIETY OF FOODS FROM ALL FIVE FOOD GROUPS HELPS YOU GROW HEALTHY AND STRONG! DRAW OR WRITE YOUR FAVORITE FOOD YOU CHOSE FROM THAT FOOD GROUP WHERE INDICATED BELOW.

	FRUIT GROUP FOODS I ATE:	VEGETABLE GROUP FOODS I ATE:	GRAIN GROUP FOODS I ATE:	PROTEIN GROUP FOODS I ATE:	DAIRY GROUP FOODS I ATE:
MONDAY DO YOUR ACTIVITES = 60 MINUTES? ☐ YES	☐☐☐☐☐ MY FAVORITE FRUIT:	☐☐☐☐☐ MY FAVORITE VEGGIE:	☐☐☐☐☐ MY FAVORITE GRAIN:	☐☐☐☐☐ MY FAVORITE PROTEIN:	☐☐☐☐☐ MY FAVORITE DAIRY:
TUESDAY DO YOUR ACTIVITES = 60 MINUTES? ☐ YES	☐☐☐☐☐ MY FAVORITE FRUIT:	☐☐☐☐☐ MY FAVORITE VEGGIE:	☐☐☐☐☐ MY FAVORITE GRAIN:	☐☐☐☐☐ MY FAVORITE PROTEIN:	☐☐☐☐☐ MY FAVORITE DAIRY:
WEDNESDAY DO YOUR ACTIVITES = 60 MINUTES? ☐ YES	☐☐☐☐☐ MY FAVORITE FRUIT:	☐☐☐☐☐ MY FAVORITE VEGGIE:	☐☐☐☐☐ MY FAVORITE GRAIN:	☐☐☐☐☐ MY FAVORITE PROTEIN:	☐☐☐☐☐ MY FAVORITE DAIRY:
THURSDAY DO YOUR ACTIVITES = 60 MINUTES? ☐ YES	☐☐☐☐☐ MY FAVORITE FRUIT:	☐☐☐☐☐ MY FAVORITE VEGGIE:	☐☐☐☐☐ MY FAVORITE GRAIN:	☐☐☐☐☐ MY FAVORITE PROTEIN:	☐☐☐☐☐ MY FAVORITE DAIRY:
FRIDAY DO YOUR ACTIVITES = 60 MINUTES? ☐ YES	☐☐☐☐☐ MY FAVORITE FRUIT:	☐☐☐☐☐ MY FAVORITE VEGGIE:	☐☐☐☐☐ MY FAVORITE GRAIN:	☐☐☐☐☐ MY FAVORITE PROTEIN:	☐☐☐☐☐ MY FAVORITE DAIRY:

Road to Health Goals:

NAME:

WEEK 3

Be active!
I intend to:

Choose
nutrient-rich foods!
I intend to:

Challenges
I might face:

Super Health Tracker

NAME:

TRACK THE DAILY SERVINGS YOU EAT FROM EACH FOOD GROUP AND LOG YOUR ACTIVITY. FINDING ACTIVITIES YOU ENJOY AND CHOOSING A VARIETY OF FOODS FROM ALL FIVE FOOD GROUPS HELPS YOU GROW HEALTHY AND STRONG! DRAW OR WRITE YOUR FAVORITE FOOD YOU CHOSE FROM THAT FOOD GROUP WHERE INDICATED BELOW.

MyPlate.gov

	FRUIT GROUP FOODS I ATE:	VEGETABLE GROUP FOODS I ATE:	GRAIN GROUP FOODS I ATE:	PROTEIN GROUP FOODS I ATE:	DAIRY GROUP FOODS I ATE:
MONDAY DO YOUR ACTIVITES = 60 MINUTES? ☐ YES	☐☐☐☐☐ MY FAVORITE FRUIT:	☐☐☐☐☐ MY FAVORITE VEGGIE:	☐☐☐☐☐ MY FAVORITE GRAIN:	☐☐☐☐☐ MY FAVORITE PROTEIN:	☐☐☐☐☐ MY FAVORITE DAIRY:
TUESDAY DO YOUR ACTIVITES = 60 MINUTES? ☐ YES	☐☐☐☐☐ MY FAVORITE FRUIT:	☐☐☐☐☐ MY FAVORITE VEGGIE:	☐☐☐☐☐ MY FAVORITE GRAIN:	☐☐☐☐☐ MY FAVORITE PROTEIN:	☐☐☐☐☐ MY FAVORITE DAIRY:
WEDNESDAY DO YOUR ACTIVITES = 60 MINUTES? ☐ YES	☐☐☐☐☐ MY FAVORITE FRUIT:	☐☐☐☐☐ MY FAVORITE VEGGIE:	☐☐☐☐☐ MY FAVORITE GRAIN:	☐☐☐☐☐ MY FAVORITE PROTEIN:	☐☐☐☐☐ MY FAVORITE DAIRY:
THURSDAY DO YOUR ACTIVITES = 60 MINUTES? ☐ YES	☐☐☐☐☐ MY FAVORITE FRUIT:	☐☐☐☐☐ MY FAVORITE VEGGIE:	☐☐☐☐☐ MY FAVORITE GRAIN:	☐☐☐☐☐ MY FAVORITE PROTEIN:	☐☐☐☐☐ MY FAVORITE DAIRY:
FRIDAY DO YOUR ACTIVITES = 60 MINUTES? ☐ YES	☐☐☐☐☐ MY FAVORITE FRUIT:	☐☐☐☐☐ MY FAVORITE VEGGIE:	☐☐☐☐☐ MY FAVORITE GRAIN:	☐☐☐☐☐ MY FAVORITE PROTEIN:	☐☐☐☐☐ MY FAVORITE DAIRY:

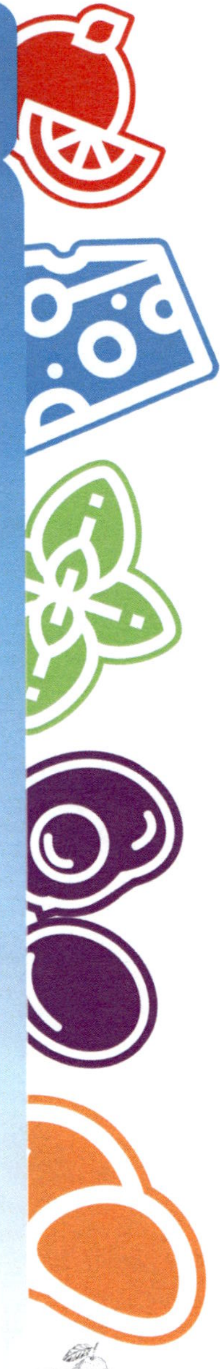

WWW.SAVOREDUCATION.COM

SAVOR EDUCATION
NUTRITION BY DESIGN

Road to Health Goals:

NAME:

WEEK 4

Be active!
I intend to:

____
____
____
____
____
____

Choose
nutrient-rich foods!
I intend to:

____
____
____
____
____
____

Challenges
I might face:

____
____
____
____
____
____

Super Health Tracker

NAME:

TRACK THE DAILY SERVINGS YOU EAT FROM EACH FOOD GROUP AND LOG YOUR ACTIVITY. FINDING ACTIVITIES YOU ENJOY AND CHOOSING A VARIETY OF FOODS FROM ALL FIVE FOOD GROUPS HELPS YOU GROW HEALTHY AND STRONG! DRAW OR WRITE YOUR FAVORITE FOOD YOU CHOSE FROM THAT FOOD GROUP WHERE INDICATED BELOW.

MyPlate.gov

	FRUIT GROUP FOODS I ATE:	VEGETABLE GROUP FOODS I ATE:	GRAIN GROUP FOODS I ATE:	PROTEIN GROUP FOODS I ATE:	DAIRY GROUP FOODS I ATE:
MONDAY DO YOUR ACTIVITES = 60 MINUTES? ☐ YES	☐☐☐☐☐ MY FAVORITE FRUIT:	☐☐☐☐☐ MY FAVORITE VEGGIE:	☐☐☐☐☐ MY FAVORITE GRAIN:	☐☐☐☐☐ MY FAVORITE PROTEIN:	☐☐☐☐☐ MY FAVORITE DAIRY:
TUESDAY DO YOUR ACTIVITES = 60 MINUTES? ☐ YES	☐☐☐☐☐ MY FAVORITE FRUIT:	☐☐☐☐☐ MY FAVORITE VEGGIE:	☐☐☐☐☐ MY FAVORITE GRAIN:	☐☐☐☐☐ MY FAVORITE PROTEIN:	☐☐☐☐☐ MY FAVORITE DAIRY:
WEDNESDAY DO YOUR ACTIVITES = 60 MINUTES? ☐ YES	☐☐☐☐☐ MY FAVORITE FRUIT:	☐☐☐☐☐ MY FAVORITE VEGGIE:	☐☐☐☐☐ MY FAVORITE GRAIN:	☐☐☐☐☐ MY FAVORITE PROTEIN:	☐☐☐☐☐ MY FAVORITE DAIRY:
THURSDAY DO YOUR ACTIVITES = 60 MINUTES? ☐ YES	☐☐☐☐☐ MY FAVORITE FRUIT:	☐☐☐☐☐ MY FAVORITE VEGGIE:	☐☐☐☐☐ MY FAVORITE GRAIN:	☐☐☐☐☐ MY FAVORITE PROTEIN:	☐☐☐☐☐ MY FAVORITE DAIRY:
FRIDAY DO YOUR ACTIVITES = 60 MINUTES? ☐ YES	☐☐☐☐☐ MY FAVORITE FRUIT:	☐☐☐☐☐ MY FAVORITE VEGGIE:	☐☐☐☐☐ MY FAVORITE GRAIN:	☐☐☐☐☐ MY FAVORITE PROTEIN:	☐☐☐☐☐ MY FAVORITE DAIRY:

WWW.SAVOREDUCATION.COM

SAVOR EDUCATION
NUTRITION BY DESIGN

Certificate of Completion
Super Health Tracker Challenge

____

Congratulations!

Made in United States
Orlando, FL
07 November 2026

90337529R00017